This book is printed in the United States of America by Joy K. Blair., No material contained in this book may be copied or retrieved in any manner for sale, but may be used in teaching and instruction for the body of Christ.

All Scripture, unless otherwise indicated, is taken from the King James Translation of the Holy Bible

Photograph by Ed Carpenter

ISBN 978-1453819166

Printed in the United States of America

Joysready34@yahoo.com

THE TRAP OF OBESITY

Transform Your Mind to Freedom

Joy Blair

Table of Contents

Dedication

I dedicate this book to my Lord and Savior Jesus Christ, to my family and to all the women who suffer with obesity and have a desire to be free from bondage to serve God with all their heart, mind, soul, and body.

Introduction

I know that being overweight can be very stressful, especially if you try to deal with it on your own without the help of God. In order to overcome this battle, you must change your mind. You don't have to live in captivity because God has set you free. He has a divine strategy for you to overcome your weight loss battle and maintain a healthy lifestyle but you must surrender to His will for your life.

I remember when hurt my back, it was an experience that I care never to repeat. While I was going through the process I learned how important it is to be in good health. I was 65 pounds or more over weight. With my back injury and the extra weight, I was very uncomfortable. Before the incident, God really began dealing with me about taking better care of my health, losing weight and getting fit for life. It's part of His covenant and His blessing for our lives.

God desires for us to be whole in every area of our lives. Until you experience sickness or any illness, it can be hard for you to appreciate good health. This is a very sentimental issue for me. I hate being overweight, it's like one of my worst nightmares. God has given me a passion for health and fitness to encourage women to be the best that they can be. I am inspired and so motivated when it comes to helping you succeed. I will go miles with you and help you press to reach your God given destination no matter how many times you need pushing.

The passion that I have is so intense because of the time I spent inside of this obesity trap just crying to come out. I know how it feels to be faced with this giant I have dealt with this overweight issue for a long time. It always made me feel inadequate and unable to perform at my 100% best. It may seem odd, but to me my life was on hold because I wasn't living the best life I knew that was mine to live.

I loved food and I made an idol out of it. I also love to exercise but I did not make it a habit. I was what you would call a seasonal disciplinarian. What I mean by this is that I would get all pumped up for a season, work out and change my eating habits and lose weight, but I would stop once I reached a certain level, never reaching my desired goal weight, just doing enough to get by.

I would only go so far as to looking a certain size to impress people but not going the nine yards for myself. I have dealt with this issue for years only because of insecurity and lack of discipline. I understood the results of having bad health habits such as eating a lot of junk foods and not exercising on a regular basis, but I practiced them anyway.

I made it a bad habit to literally put my money where my mouth was, which left me broke and overweight. I wanted to lose weight and be totally fit, but I did not want to discipline myself to get my desired results.

I remember when I first started taking diet pills, I was around 18 years old and from that point on I would always try to find some kind of diet pills to help me lose weight. The truth is the more I took the pills, after I lost the weight, the more weight I gained back.

God's desire is for us to be in good health and prosper in every area of our lives. He does not want us to depend on diet pills, having surgery or any other quick fixes. We are to practice self- control and to be led by the Holy Spirit. The LORD will lead us and guide us to make the correct decisions concerning our healthy lifestyle. We are not to depend on man for help, but on the LORD. We should make it a habit to eat healthy, workout and drink plenty of water daily and not to rush the process, but to pace ourselves with the help of God. While we are in the process of losing weight and or maintaining it we must keep God's word in our heart.

Spend time with God first every day before we do anything else. This will give you the strength you need to persevere. Make sure you do not stop putting God first once you lose the weight. You'll always need His help. This book will help you to put first things first by arranging your priorities mentally. If you change the way you think about yourself by building up your spirit man, you can bring the flesh under subjection and no longer allow it to rule over you with all its worldly gratifications and desires.

I know if you were free from obesity that you would do things that you can't even imagine. As you transform your mind you will dominate this obesity giant once and for all. It's time for you to take back your mind, health, and your life in Christ Jesus.

PRAYER FROM THE HEART

Lord I pray for every reader of this book, including myself that you help us to put you first in all that we do (Matthew 6:33) acknowledging You in everything that we do (Proverbs 3:6) and as Lord over our lives giving You full authority. Help us to understand daily that our bodies are the temple of the Holy Spirit who lives in us sent from You LORD and that we are not our own but were bought with a price. You paid the most precious price which was Your blood. Therefore help us to glorify You in our bodies and our spirit which belong to You. Help us not to make an idol out of our new healthy life style but to keep You on the throne. Help us to change all of our bad habits by practicing good healthy habits both naturally and spiritually. Father, help us to pray, study and fast so that we can be healthy & fit in the spirit growing strong and mature. Help us to eat healthy, exercise more, drink plenty of water and take our necessary vitamins and supplements so that we can be healthy and fit in the natural giving all the glory to You Lord in Jesus name. Amen.

STEP ONE

PRAYING GOD'S WORD

Be careful for nothing; but in everything by prayer and supplication with thanksgiving let your requests be made known unto God.
(Philippians 4:6)

There is all power in the Word of God. If you really understood the power that you have in the Word of God you wouldn't put it down and you definitely wouldn't take it for granted. The Word of God is eternal.

In the beginning was the Word, and the Word was with God, and the Word was God. The same was in the beginning with God. All things were made by him; and without him was not anything made that was made. And the Word was made flesh, and dwelt among us, (and we beheld his glory, the glory as of the only begotten of the Father,) full of grace and truth (John 1:1-3, 14).

Do you realize that the Word of God is God and that Jesus is the Word of God? So every time you speak God's word, which is Jesus, you literally release God in the atmosphere. This reminds me of how in the beginning God created heaven and earth. And the earth was without form, and void; and darkness was upon the face of the deep. And the Spirit of God moved upon the face of the waters. And God said, Let there be light: and there was light. And God saw the light, that it was good: and God divided the light from the darkness (Genesis 1:1-4).

The power in the word of God creates. And He has given this same power to you to do exactly what He did. Create your world with the Word of God. By speaking God's word over your life you can build your destiny and fulfill your God given purpose. With God's word you can destroy plan of Satan.

God's word is living and powerful and sharper than any two-edged sword, piercing even to the dividing asunder of soul and spirit, and of joints and marrow and is a discerner of thoughts and intents of the heart.

(Hebrews 4:12)

HIT SATAN WERE IT HURTS

The enemy always try to come and hit you where is hurts. He'll come and throw a dozen of donuts on your mind knowing that if you meditate on those donuts long enough it's just a matter of time before you'll be standing in line at the store buying them. As you stand there with that box in your hand, he tells you that either you can buy two boxes one for you and one for the family or hurry and eat the box in the car before you get home. See the captivity in his lies, instead of getting one donut and being satisfied, he wants you to suffer knowing that if you eat that whole box or even half the box, you're going to feel so guilty and not to mention that before the week is out your stomach will look like you are 9 months pregnant.

This very thing happened to me. I really don't eat donuts but one week after completing a 21 day fast, I saw some donuts that looked so good, I just had to taste one to see if they were as good as they looked.

Those donuts were so good I ate about four of them. I went back two more times that week and ate at least four donuts each time. If it wasn't for the fact that I had to share with my husband and four kids believe me I would have eaten the entire box each time.

Well by the next week my stomach was so swollen that I looked 9 months pregnant from eating all those sugary donuts. I was so embarrassed. God put me right back on a fast and this time it was for 40 days, vegetable and water only. God was using my fasts to help break off the bad habits that I had formed over the years.

I had to fast that greed demon off of me. My flesh was so strong, but God knew what I needed to humble myself. I learned to fight the devil back. When he comes to me with his tempting donuts and unhealthy foods trying to make me weak, vulnerable and depressed either because I couldn't have the food or I gave into his luring scheme, I pull out my weapon, God's word, and hit him back.

I pray God's word out loud and the enemy of our souls hates it when we mix prayer with the word of God. All of hell knows that God honors His word. Now the devil starts shaking and getting all weak, vulnerable and depressed and if that's not enough I praise God so hard until it confuse the devil and he run like a one wheel skate.

If you are going to be effective at defeating this obesity giant, than you must begin to study the Word of God. It's your weapon against the attacks of the enemy.

You are to study to show thyself approved unto God, a workman that needs not to be ashamed, rightly dividing the word of truth (2 Timothy 2:15). How can you pray the Word of God if you don't know it?

YOU'VE BEEN FAT TOO LONG

The LORD says that, you have dwelt long enough in this place it's time for you to change and go another way, the right way, God's way. I know you are tired of being fat and unhealthy and that you want change in your life. It is time for you to lose weight and begin living the life that you dream about.

This new life begins with reading, meditating, studying and praying the word of God. You will not be successful without it. God created the world with His Word and you are to create your world with God's word by declaring it over yourself.

Thou shalt also decree a thing, and it shall be established unto thee: and the light shall shine upon thy ways.

(Job 22:28)

Make God your morning joy by delighting yourself in Him and He shall give you the desires of your heart. He takes no pleasure in you worrying and being all depressed about losing weight. The more you worry the more damage you do to your body and soul. As you decide to go to God with your cares, pouring your heart out to Him, being real with God about your needs, emotions and desires you will get a release from your burden; after all, you see for yourself that all the worrying, complaining and murmuring you've done hasn't changed your weight loss process.

True rest comes from God and God alone. Take His yoke upon you and learn from Him how to be rest instead of being upset and frustrated. I remember always putting myself down saying ugly things about my weight and how much I did not like myself, as long as I would say those ungodly words I would see myself worse.

I was miserable and very unhappy. It's impossible to get any results with such a negative attitude. With that behavior, my prayers were so full of unbelief and that's why failure played such a successful role in all of my attempts. God is not going to move off your discouraged and doubtful prayers. Your attitude must be one of thanksgiving. As you thank God for who He is, what He has done and what He will do, your atmosphere will change to expectation which will build hope and give you increased confidence to ask God for anything according to His word.

God operates in the realm of faith, as you pray and thank God, His peace which can't be explained, guards your heart and mind from the trap of anxiety through Jesus Christ. Make it a habit to pray to God in faith for change because whatever is not of faith is sin (Romans 14:23). Ask Him in faith to help you to lose weight, do not put your confidence in flesh, you can't do this on your own if you could It would already have been done. God understands your need to lose weight and be healthy.

Beloved, I wish above all things that thou mayest prosper and be in health, even as thy soul prospereth.

(3 John 2)

Don't give up because you don't have your desired results pray without ceasing. I know how consuming and overwhelming you can become with being overweight. It is stressful and challenging because you feel guilty for allowing yourself to reach this level of weight gain. You don't have to live feeling condemned the Bible says that there is now no more condemnation to those who are in Christ Jesus, who do not walk in the flesh but according to the spirit (Romans 8:1).

The devil tried to trap Jesus with food, but Jesus used God's word to overpower the devil.

Then was Jesus led up of the Spirit into the wilderness to be tempted of the devil. And when he had fasted forty days and forty nights, he was afterward an hungered. And when the tempter came to him, he said, If thou be the Son of God, command that these stones be made bread. But he answered and said, It is written, Man shall not live by bread alone, but by every word that proceedeth out of the mouth of God (Matthew 4:1-4).

This is a powerful example of how the enemy will use food to ensnare you in order to keep you from your destiny. Jesus teaches us how to overcome the appetites of the flesh by fasting. Fasting prepares us for temptations and the written word of God keeps us. As long as you are trapped inside all of that weight you are no threat to the kingdom of darkness. How could you be a threat to him when you can't control your own flesh and bring it under subjection? You can't. If food has power over you, you are in the devils prison and the moment you try to cast out a demon all he has to do is wave a donut or piece of chicken and you are out for the count.

If you are going to win you must practice living a life full of discipline and God's word, it has to be more important to you than food.

Neither have I gone back from the commandment of his lips; I have esteemed the words of his mouth more than my necessary food

(Job 23:12).

Pray for the word of God to become your daily bread. You must stop thinking carnal, as long as you are in the flesh you can't please God because a carnal mind is against God, it is not subject to God and neither can it be (Romans 8:6-7). Don't worry about your life, turn it over to God and trust that the suffering that you are currently dealing with is not worthy to be compared to the glory that God has in store for you (Romans 8:18).

It's time for a shift. It's time for a change. God has a brand new life for you. Get up and fight back you can defeat this giant. Pray the word of God and be watchful to the end with all perseverance and supplication.

STEP TWO

TRANSFORM YOUR MIND WITH FASTING

And he said unto them, this kind can come forth by nothing, but by prayer and fasting.
(Mark 9:29)

Your flesh has been in control of you for years. Even though you spend all your money on food it will not satisfy your soul. To spend all your years giving in to the desires of your flesh is vanity, empty and foolish. To reach the pinnacle of your life and take a good look at yourself, the lack of loyalty, commitment and discipline to the person God has called you to be would not be a good picture.

Fasting means to abstain from physical nourishment. It is one of the greatest weapons that you have to break the yoke of bondage off your life.

Is not this the fast that I have chosen? To loose the bands of wickedness, to undo the heavy burdens, and to let the oppressed go free, and that ye break every yoke? Is it not to deal thy bread to the hungry, and that thou bring the poor that are cast out to thy house? when thou seest the naked, that thou cover him; and that thou hide not thyself from thine own flesh? Then shall thy light break forth as the morning, and thine health shall spring forth speedily: and thy righteousness shall go before thee; the glory of the LORD shall be thy rearward.

(Isaiah 58:6-8)

Adding fasting to prayer is much power. God has a chosen fast just for you, a fast that will loose you from the bondage and break the yokes that hold you captive. Your obedience determines your breakthrough to the addiction of unhealthy eating and exercise habits. Remember that fasting is a weapon and as you use it, it will break off greed and all demonic spirits.

The benefits of fasting will impact and change your life in ways you couldn't imagine both spiritual and physical. Not only will it help you to break bad eating habits but it will also help you to get rid of reoccurring sin in your life. It helps to bring your mind, will and emotion subject to the will of God because it humbles you. Fasting helps to get your prayers answered quicker. It helps to eliminate toxins, waste and allergies from your body. It helps to increase your energy and alertness.

It brings chaos and confusion to a halt allowing you to focus better and gives you more mental clarity with a sharper sense of spiritual discernment and revelation from God. Not to mention it helps you to lose weight, supercharge your health and vitality. It helps your body to heal quicker. There are so many more benefits from fasting. It is a great discipline that should be practiced by Christians not only for the benefits but out of obedience to God.

If you are willing and obedient you shall eat the good of the land.

(Isaiah 1:19).

Many people hate to hear the word fasting, because they do not want to deny the flesh any of its desires. They give in to all junk and unhealthy foods, sexual sins, fulfilling all its lust, then cry out to God when they reach a dead end. We must fast if we want to fulfill our God given purpose. It must become part of your lifestyle. Do not fast to be seen by men but to be seen by God.

> *Moreover when ye fast, be not, as the hypocrites, of a sad countenance: for they disfigure their faces, that they may appear unto men to fast. Verily I say unto you, They have their reward. But thou, when thou fastest, anoint thine head, and wash thy face; That thou appear not unto men to fast, but unto thy Father which is in secret: and thy Father, which seeth in secret, shall reward thee openly.*

> *(Matthew 6:16-18)*

DIFFERENT KINDS OF FAST

The most important benefit of fasting is to align and make your relationship right before God and to draw near to Him with all of your heart. It helps to soften your hard heart of stone, making it easier to obey and surrender to God. Fasting is also a cure for unbelief (Mark 9:29). When you are in unbelief it makes it harder to lose weight, why? Because you don't believe that you can. Why would someone pursue something that they know is impossible to obtain?

There are countless stories in the Bible on fasting and the incredible results that follow. All fasts were not the same. The best thing to do is seek God for the best fast for you. Some were *24 hour fast (2 Samuel 3:35, Nehemiah 9:1-4, 1Samuel 7:6-14)*. Some were for *3 days fast (Esther 4:13-16, Acts 9: 9, 17)*. Some fasts were *for 7 days (2 Samuel 12: 16-23, 1 Samuel 31:13)*. Some fasts were for *14 days (Acts 27: 33-34)*. There was a *21 day fast done by Daniel (Daniel 10:3)* which resulted in Daniel receiving visitation from an angel.

(Daniel 10:3-14)

I ate no pleasant bread, neither came flesh nor wine in my mouth, neither did I anoint myself at all, till three whole weeks were fulfilled. And in the four and twentieth day of the first month, as I was by the side of the great river, which is Hiddekel; Then I lifted up mine eyes, and looked, and behold a certain man clothed in linen, whose loins were girded with fine gold of Uphaz: His body also was like the beryl, and his face as the appearance of lightning, and his eyes as lamps of fire, and his arms and his feet like in colour to polished brass, and the voice of his words like the voice of a multitude. And I Daniel alone saw the vision: for the men that were with me saw not the vision; but a great quaking fell upon them, so that they fled to hide themselves. Therefore I was left alone, and saw this great vision, and there remained no strength in me: for my comeliness was turned in me into corruption, and I retained no strength. Yet heard I the voice of his words: and when I heard the voice of his words, then was I in a deep sleep on my face, and my face toward the ground. And, behold, an hand touched me, which set me upon my knees and upon the palms of my hands. And he said unto me, O Daniel, a man greatly beloved, understand the words that I speak unto thee, and stand upright: for unto thee am I now sent. And when he had spoken this word unto me, I stood trembling. Then said he unto me, Fear not, Daniel: for from the first day that thou didst set thine heart to understand, and to chasten thyself before thy God, thy words were heard, and I am come for thy words. But the prince of the kingdom of Persia withstood me one and twenty days: but, lo, Michael, one of the chief princes, came to help me; and I remained there with the kings of Persia. Now I am come to make thee understand what shall befall thy people in the latter days: for yet the vision is for many days.

Jesus fasted 40 days and 40 nights and was tempted by the devil to turn stone into bread (Matthew 4). Now if Jesus fasted and we are to walk in His footsteps, then our duty is to fast as well. Satan tempted Jesus and he will tempt you.

In order to resist the enemy and not fall for his luring temptations like Eve and Adam did, you'd better fast and pray. Absolutely too many people are giving away their God given birthright for a bowl of soup. You don't want to sell your birthright for the sake of food or anything else for that matter.

STEP THREE

WRITE THE VISION

And the LORD answered me, and said, Write the vision, and make it plain upon tables, that he may run that readeth it.
(Habakkuk 2:2)

It's time for a new vision. Pray and ask God to give you a new vision for yourself. God is ready to do a new thing for you. Remember ye not the former things, neither consider the things of old. Behold, I will do a new thing; now it shall spring forth; shall ye not know it? I will even make a way in the wilderness, and rivers in the desert. (Isaiah 43:18-19).

Don't be afraid of shifting to your next level. This level will be like nothing that you have experienced in your past.

It requires excellence and focused determination like never before. Your old dreams and plans can't compare with what God has in store for your future. But as it is written, Eye hath not seen, nor ear heard, neither have entered into the heart of man, the things which God hath prepared for them that love him (1 Corinthians 2:9).

As you pray keep a pad and pen with you expecting God to give you the new vision of yourself at your best. Write down the exact vision that you see. Next ask God to give you the plan to achieve the vision. He knows the plans that he has for you to give you the future you hope for (Jeremiah 29:11).

Once He gives you the plan, don't expect it to just appear like magic. It will take time, perseverance and hard work. I use to think that if God gave me a vision, then it was His responsibility to make it come to pass in my life. I did not realize that a dream comes by much activity (Ecclesiastes 5:3).

The vision will eventually come to pass, but you must do your part preparing for the vision, making room for it in your life. For the vision is yet for an appointed time, but at the end it shall speak, and not lie: though it tarry, wait for it; because it will surely come, it will not tarry. Behold, his soul which is lifted up is not upright in him: but the just shall live by his faith. (Habakkuk 2:3-4).

Most people give up right at the break of day. If you are going to get your desired results, you must not give up. If anyone deserves to reap the benefits of an obesity free life, then it's you.

You are the one who have to carry around all the excess baggage of fat. Your feet are the ones that are all swelled up and hurting. Why deny yourself of what is rightfully yours, a healthy and longevity life.

CONFESSION

You have everything you need right in your mouth. The devil wants to keep your mouth plugged up with food and deplete you from creating the perfect you with your words. There's power in your tongue. Begin training your tongue to work for you and not against you.

Death and life are in the power of the tongue: and they that love it shall eat the fruit thereof.

(Proverbs 18:21)

Whatever you speak out of your mouth is what you will have manifest in your life. If you continue to say that you are fat, you can't lose weight, you can't stop eating junk food, you just have to eat fast foods every day, then you will continue to have the results that you despise.

You have the ability to confess the word of God over your life and with faith filled words you will see what you believe God for come to pass in your life. (Pastor Blunt)

God is not a man that He should lie, or a son of man that He should repent has He said and will He not do? Or has He spoken, and will He not make it good (Numbers 23:19). For all the promises of God in Him are yes, and amen all we have to do is believe God God desires for us to be healthy and not sick and your words must line up with the Words of God. You must commit to be just like Jesus.

When Jesus was teaching in one of the synagogues on the Sabbath and saw a woman who had a spirit of infirmity for eighteen years and was bent over and could in no way rise herself up, Jesus called her to Him and said to her "woman you are loosed from your infirmity"

(Luke 13:10-12)

Now does that sound like a God who wants you to be sick?

Jesus only did what He saw the Father do and what the Father told Him to do (John 5:19-21).

Jesus traveled along and passed over again by ship unto the other side, much people gathered unto him: and he was nigh unto the sea. And, behold, there cometh one of the rulers of the synagogue, Jairus by name;

43

and when he saw him, he fell at his feet, And besought him greatly, saying, My little daughter lieth at the point of death: I pray thee, come and lay thy hands on her, that she may be healed; and she shall live. And Jesus went with him; and much people followed him, and thronged him. There was a certain woman, which had an issue of blood twelve years, And had suffered many things of many physicians, and had spent all that she had, and was nothing bettered, but rather grew worse, When she had heard of Jesus, came in the press behind, and touched his garment. For she said, if I may touch but his clothes, I shall be whole. And straightway the fountain of her blood was dried up; and she felt in her body that she was healed of that plague. Jesus, immediately knowing in himself that virtue had gone out of him, turned him about in the press, and said, Who touched my clothes? And his disciples said unto him, Thou seest the multitude thronging thee, and sayest thou, Who touched me? And he looked round about to see her that had done this thing. But the woman fearing and trembling, knowing what was done in her, came and fell down before him, and told him all the truth. And he said unto her, Daughter, thy faith hath made thee whole; go in peace, and be whole of thy plague

(Mark 5:21-34).

FAITH

Jesus has passion in healing His people? But without faith they would have not been healed. Faith stirs up the passion of God and release virtue from Him. Without faith you will not be set free from bondage. Our desire should be that of Jesus to care more about the will of God, healing and setting others free, than we care about food. Jesus wants you to understand that when He made you He made no mistakes. He wants you to see yourself the way that

He sees you, absolutely whole, beautiful and perfect. Don't focus on what you see when you look in the mirror, but focus on the author and finisher of your faith which is Jesus Christ. Hold your head up and walk upright you do not have to be ashamed. You must operate in the right now faith, not next week, but now. Faith is always now and its hope holds you until you receive the manifestation you desire.

Now faith is the substance of things hoped for, the evidence of things not seen. For by it the elders obtained a good report. Through faith we understand that the worlds were framed by the word of God, so that things which are seen were not made of things which do appear. But without faith it is impossible to please him: for he that cometh to God must believe that he is, and that he is a rewarder of them that diligently seek him

(Hebrews 11:1-3, 6).

You must make sure that your faith is in God and nothing else. As you put your faith in God, you will receive the faith to speak faith filled words. You build strong faith by constantly thinking, seeing, saying and believing God's word. Faith is like a coin it has two parts to it believing is the first side and speaking what you believe is the other side and if you are not saying God's word in your battle you will not win (Pastor David Blunt).

STEP FOUR

THE WHOLE ARMOR OF GOD

Put on the whole armor of God that ye may be able to stand against the wiles of the devil.
(Ephesians 6:11)

You are in a battle with the devil and he's using your flesh against you as a weapon. The battle that you are in is a fight for your life. The enemy wants to take you out of here and he's setting traps all around you in hopes to make you fall into his prey.

The same snare that he used to bait Adam and Eve and reel them in, is the same trap he tried to use on Jesus. And now he's plotting against your soul with the same *food trap*. Your job is to stand against the schemes of the devil with the whole armor of God on.

Finally, my brethren, be strong in the Lord, and in the power of his might. Put on the whole armour of God, that ye may be able to stand against the wiles of the devil. For we wrestle not against flesh and blood, but against principalities, against powers, against the rulers of the darkness of this world, against spiritual wickedness in high places. [3]Wherefore take unto you the whole armour of God, that ye may be able to withstand in the evil day, and having done all, to stand. Stand therefore, having your loins girt about with truth, and having on the breastplate of righteousness; And your feet shod with the preparation of the gospel of peace; Above all, taking the shield of faith, wherewith ye shall be able to quench all the fiery darts of the wicked. And take the helmet of salvation, and the sword of the Spirit, which is the word of God: Praying always with all prayer and supplication in the Spirit, and watching thereunto with all

perseverance and supplication for all saints;
(Ephesians 6:10-18).

We are to be strong in the Lord and in the power of His might and not in our own strength, but leaning and trusting totally in God. So many people start off running so well, they think the faster they go the quicker they'll get to their destination.

The truth about the matter is, the faster you run the quicker you become tired and weary. I remember how I use to always start off my new exercise regimen doing 6 miles a day. I would push myself so hard and when I did not see results right away, I would lose courage and become so frustrated. One day I heard the Lord say to me "pace yourself, for the race is not given to the

swift nor the battle to the strong
(Ecclesiastes 9:1) but he who endures
to the end will be saved (Matthew
10:22). Starting off trying to be supper
discipline and working yourself to hard
will only lead to failure. Yes you are to
be disciplined but you must take small
steps, one at a time.

Don't try to climb the latter by taking
all the steps at one time, you will hurt
yourself. During the battle you must
purpose in your heart that you will
stand your ground and endure. That's
right, stand your ground, don't try to
fight a battle that's not yours. Don't try
to be like no one else. Just take your
time and you will find out that it will
work out for you as it should. When
we take on too much too soon, it will

eventually cause you to quit. You will walk away from it all feeling like it's not worth it. It's worth every penny, but in proper proportion. Even in this battle to lose weight you are not wrestling against flesh and blood, but against principalities, against powers, against rulers of the darkness of this world, against spiritual wickedness in high places (Ephesians 6:12).

The devil has different methods and tactics that he use to try to deceive, enslave and ruin your life. If he can dangle something in your face to cause you to override the boundaries of God in your life he will keep using it as bait to entrap your soul. Without the armor of God on, you are vulnerable and headed for defeat. With the armor of God on, you are on the path of victory.

FACE YOUR GOLIATH

In 1 Samuel 17 David had to face Goliath because no one else would. The army was full of men of war, trained to fight the enemy. All with their fancy attire on, bows and spheres in place armed and ready for battle but afraid to stand against the giant. They were indeed ready physically, strong, tall, but mentally weak.

The battle you are facing might have been passed down to you from generation to generation. Maybe, like David, no one was bold enough to stand up against the obesity demon and now you and your children are being tormented by it. David was only 17 years old, but he had something that apparently they did not, he had faith and trust in God as his protector.

Instead of the shield that King Saul and his army used, David had the shield of faith. Though they stood there for days all afraid, David came armed and ready for the fight. It's time out for hiding from this Giant. Gird up your loins and take this bully by the throat, literally.

King Saul's army tried to do it in the flesh without God's guidance. On the other hand David was prepared because he had been in the presence of the Lord praising and worshiping God prior to the encounter with Goliath. We have to mentally prepare ourselves, by spending time with God in His Word.

David could not understand why the men of God were so afraid. He understood that the Lord was fighting on his side and the enemy did not have a winning chance. All David had physically was five smooth stones. All odds were against him, he had no great strength, height, weight or any other natural abilities. One thing he did have that the enemy did not was God on his side.

God always use the foolish thing to confuse the wise. David destroyed that giant and the bible says the others that were with the giant went fleeing different ways. God said that He will make your enemies flee from you seven different ways. They may all gang up on you at one time, but they will be running and scattered all over the place if you trust God.

Once you take this obesity giant down a lot of those other issues that you are dealing with will go as well. This is the ring leader, the head macho, the one that's causing all the trouble. Get God's word and throw it at your enemy until he is gone. God wants you to be prepared for the battle. His desire is for you to conquer this giant one stone at a time, just like David did destroying it once and for all never dealing with this one again. Imagine the freedom. You can't be lazy or naïve in protecting yourself, only putting on certain pieces of armor. The devil will be shooting at every angle. You are to put the whole armor on for yourself and don't expect no one else to cover you it's your responsibility if you want to stand and not fall in the evil days of temptation.

Never be caught off guard sleeping when you should be standing. It's time to wake up out of your sleep to righteousness and do not sin. You are to be self controlled and watchful because your adversary the devil walks about like a roaring lion seeking whom he may devour (1 Peter 5:8). Obesity is not just about your body not being attractive. It's more than you being able to fit into your skinny jeans. It's warfare.

It's a struggle with the power of darkness and the forces they operate with to keep us from the land that God has promised you which includes a healthy life, free from obesity. You are on the battlefield rather you understand it or not. Your enemy knows that you are enlisted in God's militant operation.

Your best bet is to get ready for battle by renewing your mind in God's word (Romans 12:2) because it's coming ready or not.

STEP FIVE

FOCUS

Looking unto Jesus the author and finisher of our faith; who for the joy that was set before him endured the cross, despising the shame, and is set down at the right hand of the throne of God. (Hebrews 12:2)

No matter the opposition Jesus did not take His eyes off the prize. What was the prize that had Jesus so focused and daring under all the pressure? You got it, you and me. We were the joy that was set before Him. He despised all the shame, lies and distractions of the enemy all the way to the cross, ascending from the grave and all the way back to the throne of

God. Make this your motivation. Jesus took all the brutal pain and suffering so that you can live a life of victory in every area of your life.

Forget about how big your legs are and go walking. I remember when I would go walking at the park and seeing other people I would feel ashamed because of how big I was. I would be so tempted to just leave and go home. It felt like everybody was watching the fat girl. Don't settle for excuses.

Your job is to get the plan from God and carry it out till the end. Don't look to your left or your right but focus on your goal. Keep your plan in your face and let nothing come between it. I know how easy it is to get distracted that's the purpose for this chapter. Focus is the only way you will ever reach any destination in life. There will be things that are designed to come against you to keep you from shifting but that's what makes change so valuable, you embraced every moment, you stood your ground and did not give up and that's what enables you to say boldly "I can do all things through Christ that strengthens me" (Philippians 4:13).

DETERMINATION

You must be determined to reach your goal. I once read a poster that said "A man can succeed at almost anything for which he has unlimited enthusiasm". I'll add to that statement, "In Jesus Christ". I know that without God we can do absolutely nothing (John 15:5). Dr. Juanita Bynum say's "One Focus". Bishop Jakes say's "Single Hearted". Jesus says' "A house divided cannot stand" (Luke 11:14).

Therefore not to be focused is to miss your target because you are aiming in the wrong place. No focus equals confusion and God is not the author of confusion. We are to keep our eyes on our prize, not looking back. Why do we take our eyes off the things we desire, to look back on things that we hate? Forget those things behind you and reach toward those things ahead of you to obtain your prize (Philippians

3:13-14). If you keep looking back, you are going to go back. We are to lay aside every weight and the sin that so easily catches us up and cause us to get off focus. If you set your focus on your ideal weight then when the tempter comes along tempting you to eat something that's not part of your healthy food list you can stand your ground and not fall for his trap and eventually reach your goal. You are to be so focused nothing can penetrate through your lens.

DESTINATION

To focus is to be determined to reach your goal cutting away everything that try to stop you from reaching it.

There's a story in the Bible in the book of Luke 19:1-10 about a man by the name of Zacchaeus who was a chief tax collector and a very rich man. He heard that Jesus had entered the town and that He was coming his way. He sought to see this Jesus that he had heard so much about but he could not because of all the people crowded around for he was a very short man.

Instead of him just setting there feeling sorry for himself, he was so determined to see Jesus that he climbed up into a sycamore tree. This man did not let anything stop him from his destination. When Jesus passed by He saw Zacchaeus up in that tree and was so moved by his persistent faith that He told him to come down from the tree and let's go to your house for dinner. This man's focus and determination caused him to not only reach his destination, but to have Destiny reach him, now that's powerful. The only thing that should be able to get your attention is the things that are part of your assignment, anything else should be considered trash so just pitch it.

STEP SIX

DISCIPLINE

But I keep under my body, and bring it into subjection: lest that by any means, when I have preached to others, I myself should be a castaway.
(1 Corinthians 9:27)

The *Greek* word for *discipline* is *sophronismos* from the word *sophron* meaning *"saving the mind"; primarily, and admonishing or calling to soundness of mind, or to self control.* You are in a race and of course you want to win. In order to win and receive your prize of losing weight and overcoming obesity you must practice discipline. The good news about discipline is that it is one of the fruit of the Holy Spirit. The not so good news is that you must develop it. This means you have some work to do.

But the fruit of the Spirit is love, joy, peace, longsuffering, gentleness, goodness, faith, Meekness, temperance: against such there is no law.

(Galatians 5:22-23)

God has placed within each of us everything that we need to accomplish our assignments and live a successful and fulfilling life in Him. If you want to reach your ideal weight and live a healthy lifestyle, and I know you do, you must be temperate in all things.

Losing weight will take months of severe training and dedication. As you fight, fight with assurance that you will win. Give no place to laziness or sloth. When you feel laziness trying to slow you down, overcome by going the extra mile, do more then you were planning on doing. Your body will try to dominate, rule and reign over you.

You are to keep your body under subjection to you. Fight like never before with discipline in your every blow. The fight that you are fighting is with yourself a war against your flesh and spirit. Your spirit wants to do the right thing but your flesh does not. Your flesh is your enemy and you must see it for what it is.

Stop giving in to its evil desires, keep it under by denying it the right to control you and order you around with its sinful gratifications. Your body must become your slave and obey you. This is a long life process. Your flesh will never be satisfied no matter how much you give in to it. That's why the Bible tells us to Love not the world, neither the things that are in the world. If any man loves the world, the love of the Father is not in him. For all that is in the world, the lust of the flesh, and the lust of the eyes, and the pride of life, is not of the Father, but is of the world (1 John 2:15-16).

You can overcome any temptation because greater is He that is in you than He that is in the world (1John 4:4). It is your job to discipline your body and not God's job. He is with you to help you but you must take the necessary steps. It's time to become serious about your weight loss, you can do it.

COMMITMENT

If you want to lose weight, you have to be committed. Thanks to God I have had the opportunity to pray, encourage and exercise with women and at the same time experiencing spiritual growth. I have always had a passion for helping women overcome life obstacles especially losing weight mostly because of the struggle I have had with being overweight.

If you keep pushing forward and stay committed you will see results. One beautiful young lady that I had the opportunity to meet really inspired me. She was extremely overweight and very discouraged about her weight problem. We decided to meet every morning at 5:00am at the local college to walk. Our goal was to make sure we put God first, so we committed to get up earlier in order to spend time with God alone before we met to walk. We were so grateful to God for His presence. He honored both of our commitments. We would pray every morning together and make our confessions as we walked encouraging each other. As time passed we begin to see results. I loved watching her emerge from being so low and discouraged to motivating and committed. The more you keep going the easier it becomes and the more you will grow to really enjoy your exercise time.

Make it a time of praising and thanking God. Giving Him the glory for everything He has done for you. Thank Him for the activity of your limbs. Don't complain but be grateful. Your attitude has a great deal to do with your results. If you are always negative and complaining you will not last too long. Keep a positive attitude by meditating on God.

This book of the law shall not depart out of thy mouth; but thou shalt meditate therein day and night, that thou mayest observe to do according to all that is written therein: for then thou shalt make thy way prosperous, and then thou shalt have good success.
(Joshua 1:8)

My friend started out discouraged and looking at her situation and as long as she remained in that state of mind nothing moved for her. As she made a decision to put God first and trust Him for His help she was encouraged and not long after she began seeing her desired results.

God is with you and He will never leave you. And because God is with you, you will overcome and reach your desired weight loss goals and help others to overcome as well.

Commit to a life of prayer and studying God's word. Choose to put Him first and He will give you the strength to persevere and endure. Change the way you eat. Stop eating out all of the time wasting your money and then complaining about being broke. Limit your intake of greasy foods and cut junk food all the way down and cut sugar out of your diet. These foods make your body swell. Eat more fruit, vegetables and baked or grilled chicken, fish or turkey and you will feel the difference in your body.

Eat healthy at least 5 days a week and have maybe one or two days for foods that are not part of your plan. That way you won't deprive yourself of certain foods that you really like and fall back into bad habits.

The purpose is to find a plan that fit you so that you can build new healthy habits instead of the bad habits you are use too. Once you see the difference in your body, mind and spirit, it will drive you to want to do the right thing for your health. Heavy and unhealthy foods weigh down your spirit.

The less you eat the more you can hear from God. Practice eating smaller portions, this will help your stomach to shrink. It is not a sin for you to eat unhealthy but you must understand that everything is not helpful for your body. Leave all those fruit juices and sweet drinks alone and replace it with water. Your body is made up of at least 70% water. In order for you to lose weight the healthy way you must drink plenty of water. Water is the source for a long and healthy life. You should be drinking at least half your body weight. If you weight 150 lbs. then you need to drink a little more than half a gallon of water a day (75 ounces).

It's also important to take vitamins and mineral supplements daily to help give your body the additional nutrients that's needed. Adding on a good protein shake is very profitable or even a fruit smoothie with protein in it is very healthy and tasty. Choose the right exercise program fit for you. Keep it simple don't try to start off with big steps, pace yourself. Your body will let you know how far to go. As you are faithful in the small steps your body will be able to tolerate more and your desire for more will increase.

Always remember every bit of exercise counts. I lost some of the most weight by walking 15-30 minutes a day. Take your time and be committed to your regimen and watch the weight fall off your mind, body and spirit. Let me make something very clear to you. Your flesh is going to always try to run things, but you have the power to win. Cast the old nature down and walk in the newness of life.

STEP SEVEN

USE EVERYTHING YOU GOT

And we know that all things work together for good to them that love God, to them who are the called according to his purpose.
(Romans 8:28)

This is the final step to transforming your mind to freedom. It involves taking every step and putting them all together for great success. In the first step we have Praying Gods Word. If you take time to get to know God through His word you'll get a better understanding of praying the word of God.

The bible says that God sent His word to heal us and to deliver us from all our destructions (Psalm 107:20) and it also says that His word will not return to Him void but it will accomplish what He please and prosper in the thing for which He sent it to do (Isaiah 55:11).

It also says that God is not a man that He should lie or a son of man that He should repent. Has He said and will He not do? Or has He spoken and will He not make it good? (Numbers 23:19) Put God's word to work for you.

Second you have fasting. Fasting is so vital. This obesity demon is very stubborn and the bible says that some demons will not leave except by prayer and fasting (Mark 9:29). Adding fasting to your prayer life is double jeopardy, power point winning tools.

The third part is to write the vision. This is so important because it's a destination map. It is the place where you desire to be. You must write it down and keep it before your face. This will help inspire you and keep you from getting discouraged while you are working toward your goal. The dream may seem as though it is not reachable and the devil will do everything possible to steal it from you, but it is yours. Look at it every day and declare that it will come to pass in your life.

The fourth step is putting on the whole armor of God. This includes seven vital pieces that will enable you to sand against the enemy in battle. Stand therefore, having your loins girded about with truth, and having on the breastplate of righteousness; And your feet shod with the preparation of the gospel of peace; Above all, taking the shield of faith, wherewith ye shall be able to quench all the fiery darts of the wicked. And take the helmet of salvation, and the sword of the Spirit, which is the word of God & pray without ceasing (Ephesians 6:14-17).

The fifth step is focus. Adding focus to the first four steps will ensure you victory. As you plant your eyes on your target and press in with all your heart you will achieve your dream. The sixth step is discipline. Implementing discipline is a sure way to eliminate self destruction.

The more you practice self control the more power you gain in battle. As you take and apply all these steps you will overcome the mental road blocks hindering you from your ideal weight. As you transform your mind, you will see clearly the power you have over obesity and get rid of it forever.

PRAYER OF SALVATION

If you have never asked Jesus into your life as your Lord and Savior now is the perfect time. He is waiting with open arms. The Bible says in Romans 10:9-10 that if you shalt confess with your mouth the Lord Jesus, and shalt believe in your heart that God hath raised Him from the dead, thou shalt be saved. For with the heart man believeth unto righteousness; and with the mouth confession is made unto salvation.

Just repeat after me.

Lord Jesus I confess with my mouth and believe in my heart that you are Lord and that you died on the cross for my sins and rose again on the third day for me. Come into my heart and fill me with Your Holy Spirit.

If you made a decision for Christ today welcome into our family ask God to lead and guide you to a church home so that you can be trained how to live life as a victorious Christian. God bless you.

Joy K Blair is married to Gregory Blair Sr. She has four beautiful children. She's an evangelist, Bible teacher, author and poet. She lives in St Louis Missouri with her family. She loves to use her multiple gifts to build up the body of Christ. She loves to motivate and inspire women to birth out their dreams for Jesus Christ.

She can be reached by email at

Joysready34@yahoo.com

By mail at

P O Box 303 Florissant Mo 63032

THE TRAP OF OBESITY